FITNESS AND FINANCE

FITNESS AND FINANCE

How to Manage your Health and Wealth

TRE FIT

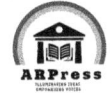

Copyright © 2021 by Tre Fit

All rights reserved. No part of this publication may be reproduced, distributed, or transmitted in any form or by any means, including photocopying, recording, or other electronic or mechanical methods, without the prior written permission of the copyright owner and the publisher, except in the case of brief quotations embodied in critical reviews and certain other noncommercial uses permitted by copyright law. For permission requests, write to the publisher, addressed "Attention: Permissions Coordinator," at the address below.

The author of this book advises to consult with a financial advisor before making any financial decisions. And before starting any exercise or nutrition program, the author advises to consult with your doctor to get clearance. The intent of the author is to offer information that may help you in your journey in physical health and wealth. In any event you use any of the information in this book for yourself, the author and publisher assume no responsibility for your actions.

ARPress
45 Dan Road Suite 5
Canton MA 02021

Hotline: 1(800) 220-7660
Fax: 1(855) 752-6001

Ordering Information:
Quantity sales. Special discounts are available on quantity purchases by corporations, associations, and others. For details, contact the publisher at the address above.

Printed in the United States of America.

ISBN-13:	Paperback	979-8-89389-830-9
	eBook	979-8-89389-831-6

Library of Congress Control Number: 2024923507

CONTENTS

Preface 1
Acknowledgments 3
Wealth 5
Health 11

Chapter 1 15
    Personal Finance 15

Chapter 2 19
    Starting a Healthy Lifestyle 19
    Assessment 20
    Not Sticking to the Program 21
    Being Impatient 22
    Health Issues 24
    Giving Up 25

Chapter 3 27
    Financial Literacy 27
    Financial Management 28
    Save 10% of Your Income 31
    Budgeting 31
    Ways to Increase Your Income 32
    Getting Rid of Bad Debt (Trimming the Fat) 33
    Understanding Credit And Credit Score 33
    Investing in the Stock Market 36

Chapter 4 41
    Diet and Exercise 41
    Body Fat Range For Women and Men 43
    Skeletal Muscle Range for Women and Men 44
    BMI Range 45
    Visceral Fat Levels 46
    Macronutrients Carbs, Protein and Fats 46
    Carbohydrates 47
    Protein 47
    Fats 47
    Exercising 48

Chapter 5 53
    Managing and Maintaining Your Health and Fitness .. 54
    Managing and Maintaining Your Wealth 55

About the Author 61

PREFACE

The purpose of this book is to provide information that may help you improve your lifestyle in fitness and personal finance. By studying this book you are investing in learning about health and wealth. If you're struggling to balance both your health and wealth this book is a great guide to help you to balance both within your lifestyle.

Having a passion for health and fitness, I became a certified NASM CPT and Precision nutrition coach, to help people improve their lifestyle through health and fitness. Since becoming a fitness coach 9 years ago, I've helped plenty of people get into shape, and some have lost up to 100 pounds! My passion for fitness led me to become passionate about personal finance. The more I learned about personal finances, I started to realize that personal finance was a topic plenty of people struggle with, just like health, and fitness. Both topics require a plan to get to your goal. In this book you will see the correlation between health and wealth. The key is to learn how to balance them within your lifestyle. Most people I know want to be healthy and wealthy. After reading this book, it should provide you with the knowledge to improve your lifestyle in health and wealth. My life changed when I focused on balancing my health, and wealth, and if I can do it, you can too. Like the saying goes "health is wealth".

ACKNOWLEDGMENTS

I want to acknowledge all of my clients from the past to present. Every one of you inspired me in one way or another, and without that inspiration, I wouldn't be where I am today. And to acknowledge everyone that is taking their time out to read this book. I appreciate your support and I'm sending you plenty of blessings in your pursuit in health and wealth.

WEALTH

> *"The road to success is always under construction"*
> **Lily Tomlin**

What is your definition of wealth? Take some time to think about it. According to Google, wealth can be categorized into three principal categories: personal property, including homes or automobiles; monetary savings, such as the accumulation of past income; and the capital wealth of income producing assets, including real estate, stocks, bonds, and businesses. Having wealth isn't only about being rich, there is more to it than that. Wealth is also having the freedom to do whatever you want to do, whenever you want to do it, without worrying how it's going to get done. Acquiring wealth is more than making money, it means different things to different people from physical wealth, emotional wealth and financial wealth as well.

Have you ever heard the term "paper chasing or chasing the bag". The term refers to making money. I personally don't use the terminology, because when you think about the term on a deeper level, when you are chasing something, it's running away from you. So you have to put in all this effort to "chase" it. And it's not guaranteed you're going to catch it. So instead of "chasing the bag" the goal is to "acquire the bag". When you think about the people who have acquired wealth, they are not "chasing the bag". They are acquiring investment assets. If your goal in life is to one day become wealthy, you're going to have to create a financial plan to make that happen. One of the keys for you to make that happen, is you're going to have to invest in assets that will bring in passive income, this is one of the keys to building wealth. When it comes to investing most people, say investing seems difficult, and even stressful, and they would rather not get into it. In a recent study 43% of people aged 25 to 34, said they weren't investing in stocks, bonds, or real estate. Most said they didn't feel as though they had enough money to start investing, they also feared losing money in the stock market, or they found investing to be complicated and intimidating, but what they don't know, is that not getting invested early, they are sacrificing the two most important things when it comes to building wealth from investing in the stock market, time, and compound interest.

Learning how to build wealth is not something that is taught in grade school. So how do we learn how to build wealth? First invest in your education, and learn about the asset you are interested in investing in. It is always a wise choice to invest in your education. Just by reading this book right now you're investing your education. Having the knowledge and then applying it, is how you get to the next level in life. Once you're educated in any field, no one can take that from you. There is a saying that goes "the more you learn, the more you earn". As young kids we are taught to be employees and consumers, and to participate in the rat race. According to wikipedia, the definition of the rat race is, "the rat race is an endless, self-defeating, or pointless pursuit. The term equates to rats attempting to earn a reward such as cheese, in vain. It may also refer to a competitive struggle to get ahead financially or routinely". So early in life we strive for our dream job, dream home and dream car. All of that is fine, except working a 9-5 job to acquire those things will be a struggle for most people. In order to acquire those things and not struggle to get them, you'll have to have multiple streams of income. And the best way to get multiple streams of income is to invest in assets that will bring you passive income. A 9-5 job is active income. Active income is considered any income that requires your time. Another source of income is passive or residual income. Passive income is any income that doesn't require your time. So the goal is to have an active and passive income stream while you are on the road to building wealth. The average millionaire has 7 streams of income. The key here is to find ways to increase your income streams. Trading hours for dollars is the long road to wealth.

In a recent CNBC article 63% of people are living paycheck to paycheck, especially since the covid-19 pandemic. As of this writing the unemployment rate is at 6.2 percent, and the number of unemployed people is at 10.0 million, this has changed little in February 2021. Although both measures are much lower than their April 2020 highs, they remain well above their pre-pandemic levels in February 2020 (3.5 percent and 5.7 million, respectively).

Investment assets are the best form of passive income. What is considered an investment asset. Some people are confused as to what is considered an investment asset. At one point I was too. The simple answer is an investment asset is any investment that brings back a return on that initial investment. So if you buy a home or car and neither is bringing in any income then that is considered a liability. It is not an asset. What is a liability? It's the opposite of an asset. It's an investment that doesn't bring any return from that investment. And this rule doesn't only apply in finance, it applies to all aspects of your life. You can have friends and family members who are more of a liability than an asset. If you have friends and family that isn't helping you get to the next level mentally, physically, financially and spiritually then you need to find new friends who can uplift you in those areas. Learn to focus your time and energy in building and maintaining your assets and get rid of and limit your liabilities. In the book the Millionaire next door, one of the key points I got from the book was "one of the foundations to wealth is through real estate." When you buy a home and rent it out that is when your home is considered an asset or when you sell it for a profit. With having investment real estate, you can get rental income every month, and this is one of the fastest ways to build wealth, for one, you can get monthly rental income from the property, and every month you pay your mortgage you're building equity in the property at the same time. That's just one way to create passive income when you're on your road to building wealth, there are several other streams of passive income you can build, you can start a business, invest in the stock market, start an online store, just to name a few. You have to get started and do what works for you. When it comes to building wealth you have to be willing to sacrifice a lot of things, so that you can put more of your wealth towards investments that are right for you. Delayed gratification is what true wealth builders live by. They live modestly and spend less than they can afford, so that they are able to invest for the future. When it comes to delayed gratification, that is one of the biggest hindrances to wealth building. Because most people want to put the horse before the carriage. Here's an example, some people want to look wealthy instead of actually being wealthy. Having a luxury car that you have to pay for out of pocket every month is actually decreasing your wealth. The goal is to create investment assets that will pay for that luxury car. So it would be wise to sacrifice on the front end, so you don't have to worry about how you're going to pay for your luxuries on the back end. We all know it takes discipline to maintain your wealth. In order to become successful you must have a success mindset. The first step to success, is you have to come up with a plan for success. The next step is to take action. When you start your day, start it with saying, I'm going to get physically fit, and then take action. Same goes for your wealth. Start your day with, I'm going to become wealthy and take action. No one can expect to change overnight. But you can take small steps towards your goals. Change can be hard because we tend to resist change. That's because when you're used to doing the same thing over and over it becomes easy and comfortable. When you have to change your routine or lifestyle it can be a struggle in the beginning because everything you're going to do is new to you. Remember if it was easy everyone would be doing it. All you have to do is set small goals for yourself and get started. No one has lost 100 pounds overnight, just like no one became rich overnight, unless they hit the lotto.

HEALTH

> *"If you take care of the small things,
> the big things take care of themselves"*
> **Emily Dickinson**

Do you know the definition of physical health? It is the result of regular exercise, proper diet and nutrition, and proper rest for physical recovery. A person who is physically fit will be able to walk or run without getting breathless and they will be able to carry out the activities of everyday living and not need help. In today's society being healthy and wealthy is one of the greatest gifts to have. We all know someone who is healthy, but not necessarily wealthy, and someone is wealthy, but not necessarily healthy. Like the saying goes "health is wealth" and "wealth is health."

Less than a quarter of Americans are meeting all national physical activity guidelines, from the Centers for Disease Control and Prevention's National Center for Health Statistics (NCHS). Federal physical activity guidelines recommend that adults get at least 150 minutes of moderate or 75 minutes of vigorous exercise each week, in addition to muscle strengthening activities at least twice a week.

But according to the new NCHS report, which drew on five years of data from the National Health Interview Survey, only about 23% of adults ages 18 to 64 are hitting both of those marks. Another 32% met one but not both, and almost 45% did not hit either benchmark.

We all know someone who needs to live a healthier lifestyle through diet and exercise, but refuse to take action. I personally have a few friends. When I ask some of them about living a healthy lifestyle, the common answer I hear is "I'm going to die from something one day." This answer is quite puzzling to me. Even after going to get a physical check up from a doctor, who recommended that they change their diet, and start an exercise program, they still refuse to take action on living a healthy lifestyle. But why? My guess is that the will to get started is not strong enough. Only when something major happens with their health is when they take it seriously. But that could have been avoided if they just changed their diet and started exercising.

Some of the people I've assessed with health issues, will say I can't afford a fitness coach. At that point, I would say, you can't afford not to have one. Physical health is not a luxury but a lifestyle to invest in. When someone prioritizes investing in their physical health, being able to afford a fitness coach will not be an issue. I usually explain to them that hiring a fitness coach is an investment in their physical health. And my job as a fitness coach is to educate, and teach them everything they need to know for them to reach their health and fitness goals, but it's their job to apply it.

When it comes to illnesses like diabetes, heart disease, and cardiovascular disease, these diseases are preventable and reversible, only if people choose to live a healthier lifestyle through a balanced diet, and exercise. This is why you should invest in your physical health on the front end so you don't have to pay for it on the back end with health issues, doctor visits, medications and time off of work, all these issues take away from your well being.

One of the things I've noticed, as a fitness coach, is that some people don't prioritize their health. Some people will work hard at a job that they might not like, that can be causing them stress and they will prioritize their job more than prioritizing their physical health. When you neglect your physical health it shortens your lifespan.

During some of my health, and fitness consultations, I would ask clients about their eating habits throughout the day. Some people will tell me that they will go to the local deli, Starbucks to name a few to get breakfast. And breakfast sometimes consists of a latte, bagel, egg and cheese sandwich, and even donuts. None of these are really healthy, not to mention nutritionally balanced. This is why investing in a dietitian or nutritionist is very important because most people are not following the basic nutritional guidelines. Being educated in nutrition will help you make better eating decisions. For some people depending on the job would not eat for hours or not at all. As a fitness coach, I would remind clients that this is not healthy, when you're starving yourself, you are at risk of fainting and passing out. This can affect job performance and can cause serious injury. Starving yourself is just as bad as eating unhealthy. Later, I will show you how to come up with solutions to tackle these issues. As a fitness coach I've conducted thousands of health, and fitness assessments with people from all walks of life, and economic backgrounds. One thing for sure, everyone I assessed wanted to get started on living a healthier lifestyle. For some people getting started is a challenge, because it requires behavioral change. Research has shown that behavioral changes can be difficult. Especially, when it comes to diet and exercise. Going from eating fast food every day to now cooking your own foods can be a challenge. Just like going from being a couch potato to now getting up every day to go for a run or hitting the gym. The key here is to just get started and start slow. Set small goals, then work towards bigger ones. In no time this will become a regular part of your lifestyle.

You have one life and one body. Your health and wealth should be the number one priority. Can you imagine, you have all the wealth you need, but you're not healthy enough to enjoy it. If you're not making health, and wealth a priority in your life, you're doing a disservice to you and your family.

CHAPTER 1

> *"Life is a marathon, not a sprint"*
> Phillip C. McGraw

PERSONAL FINANCE

When it comes to personal finance, we all strive for financial stability. Having financial stability is less stressful than living paycheck to paycheck. The covid-19 pandemic of 2020 is a perfect example, as to why financial stability is very important. Millions of people lost their jobs, overnight due to the government shut down, including myself. While the government did give us aid, depending where you live in the USA, it wasn't enough for places like NYC, where everything is more expensive than the average city across the USA. The unemployment rate is at an all-time high, and at the same time, millions of households are facing evictions, businesses are closing down, and home owners are facing foreclosures. No one predicted something like this could ever happen. I only saw this in movies, and here we are living it out in real time. This should be a learning lesson to all, that we have to always work towards building wealth by investing in assets that will bring in multiple sources of income. So when times like these happen we are better prepared.

I want to tell you a story about one of my childhood friends. Tony is a childhood friend I grew up with since I was 5 years old. We grew up as cousins, so my mom was his aunt, just like his mom was my Aunt even though we weren't really related. When we would do sleep overs, I liked sleeping at his house because he had all the toys and video games. His mom made sure he had all the latest toys and video and the latest clothes so he looked good at all times. Because he was an only child his mom took good care of him. Once we became adults, Tony went on to work at DSNY, which is the department of sanitation in NYC. He started young and was making a decent income. Even though he was making a decent income, he only relied on that one source income. He started living above his means and this is where he went wrong, he was more concerned with driving a luxury car and dressing flashy instead of working towards building wealth during his working years. I have to admit, I got caught up in buying high end clothes too, but only when I could afford it. What he didn't take into consideration was now he is working a 9-5 job to maintain his lifestyle, trading hours for dollars. He didn't want to downgrade his image, so he maintained that image, until it put him in a financial bind. Once his expenses became too high things got over his head. He was carrying a lot of debt and fixed expenses. Here is the list of debt and fixed expenses he was carrying. 1) Very high credit card debt, 2) two personal loans, 3) store cards, 4) car note, 5) car insurance, 6) life insurance, 7) health insurance, 8) phone bill, 9) child support, 10) cable, and 11) rent. These are just the major fixed debt and expenses he had. With all that debt and expenses, it put him in a financial bind. His expenses were higher than his income. His debt to income ratio was way off balance. His debt was too high and he needed to cut all the bad debt, so he could balance his debt to income ratio.

So let me tell you what happened next. He was paying off all his debt and fixed expenses, but because he wasn't making enough money, he was neglecting to pay his rent. I asked him why he would do that.

He told me he did this because he didn't want to ruin his credit score and default on any of the loans or credit cards. He said if he defaulted on the car loan it would get repossessed and if he defaulted on any loans or credit cards it would negatively affect his credit score. So he was willing to sacrifice paying his rent, to pay off his bad debt and expenses first. He explained to me having a good credit score is very important. Eventually his rent backed up to a point where he had to go to eviction court. In February 2020 he went to court to resolve the issue. He was backed up $3,200 plus the current months' rent, which brought it to $4,500.

When he went to court he spoke to the rental property lawyer, the lawyer asked him how he wanted to resolve the issue. Tony told him he understands that he owes that much money, so he plans on paying it. The lawyer then asked how long he needed to pay it off. He said he'll have it by the end of the month. He told me the lawyer was surprised he said that, and the lawyer said ok, but if it's not paid by the end of the month, they will proceed with the eviction. He said no problem. This was February 5th, and we know February is the shortest month of the year. I let him know that the first thing he has to do is increase his income ASAP. He let me know he wasn't looking for any handouts, because he got himself in that mess, and it was his responsibility to get out. So what I suggested was for him to get a side hustle with a delivery service. He did have a vehicle, so I told him he could utilize it to do delivery work to help increase his income.

He was very happy to be doing this side hustle. This side hustle was bringing him in an extra $500-$600 per week. And this was what he did to increase his income. And by the end of the month he paid off the rent and the eviction case was dropped. He later told me that was a learning lesson for him. I told him he has to live within his means and get out of the rat race mentality. I told him he should read "Rich Dad Poor Dad" by Robert Kiyosaki and Sharon Lechter. I personally like that book because it tells you the difference between an asset and liability. My friend Tony only spent his money on liabilities and didn't have any assets. After he read the book he told me he wished he would have read it years ago, because he would have known the difference between an asset and liabilities and have a better understanding on how to utilize his money. The lesson he learned was not to get into bad debt for materialistic things, but instead get assets that will grow in value over time. One big thing he also learned was his car was a liability, until he started using it to bring in an income. Using his car to do deliveries made the car become an asset.

I also told him to speak with a "personal financial coach" who will help him understand how to manage his finances better. One thing he learned about bad debt is that it's like body fat, it's there, and seems like it isn't going anywhere. That's why you don't want to get there in the first place. Especially, if you just pay the minimum every month on a high interest loan or credit card. You'll be paying it back for a very long time, especially if your credit cards are maxed out. Now you can see how this relates to fat loss. If you do the minimum amount of work, it's going to take a long time to lose the fat. I wanted to share this story to show you how bad debt can set you back financially if not managed right. It's okay to seek help before it's too late.

When looking at bad debt, it's not bringing any income in return, so it's a liability. Example, a car you're making monthly payments on, that's not making you any money in return. My friend Tony turned his car to an asset when he started using it to do delivery work to increase his income.

CHAPTER 2

> *"The price of success is hard work, dedication to the job at hand and the determination that, whether we win or lose, we have applied the best of ourselves to the task at hand"*
> **Vincent Lombardi**

STARTING A HEALTHY LIFESTYLE

When it comes to starting a healthy lifestyle, it can be a challenge, especially if you have no experience in dieting and exercise. That's why it is important to seek out a fitness coach who can guide you through the process of reaching your fitness goals. My job as a fitness coach is to find out what your goals are, and come up with a plan for you to reach them. One thing I do ask a client before we get started, is "why" do they want to get started now, this is a very important question to ask. I want to know "why" you want to start this lifestyle change. Asking "why" is very important because this is their motivating factor as to why they are there to see me in the first place. Everyone has a different "why". Some of the most common reasons I hear is, the doctor recommended it, getting married, just had a recent break up, wants to get healthy, going on a vacation and other reasons.

ASSESSMENT

One of the first things I'll do with a potential client is a PARQ. This is the Physical Activity Readiness Questionnaire (**PAR-Q**) is a common method of uncovering health, and lifestyle issues, prior to starting an exercise program. The questionnaire is short and easy to administer, and reveals any family history of illness. In some cases if a person has health issues they will have to get an approval from their doctor to start an exercise program. Once that's out the way I'll take their physical stats. Weight, BMI, body fat, muscle mass, body age, metabolic rate, and visceral fat. After reviewing the stats with them, sometimes I've noticed some of the people would start to take their health more seriously, especially if the stats were not good. Something else that's very important, when starting an exercise program is pictures for seeing the visual progression. With these stats, and pictures, you can keep track to see if you're progressing.

After that is done we'll talk about their current diet. This is where I get a lot of push back, because some people are used to eating a certain way. I've done assessments with people across all cultural backgrounds, and one of the common things I would here is I'm from India, so we eat like this, I'm west Indian, so we eat like this, I'm from the south, so we eat like this, you get the point. So diet is connected to all cultural backgrounds. And getting people to change that can be a challenge for any fitness coach. I let them know that in order to reach their fitness goal the diet must change.

I'll explain to them that 80% is diet and 20% is exercise, when it comes to reaching their fitness goals. So eating healthy is a very important part of the puzzle. I would also give them a nutritional guideline to follow, which consists of good carbs, protein, and fats to eat, while on their fitness program.

The next part of the assessment is where I'll do a physical assessment of the person. I'll have them perform a few exercises like squats, pushups, planks, and 1 minute of step ups or bicycle. This is done to determine their fitness level, so I can know what level they should start. Once that's done we'll sit, and go over the physical assessment, and talk about where some improvement can be made. There are all types of physical conditions people are not aware of. That's why the assessment is important. I've come across people who think they're physically fit, but are not. I'll have someone stand on one leg for 30 seconds, and believe it or not some people can't. Or even hold a plank position, some people can't hold a plank position for 30 seconds, and most people squat wrong. The key to squatting is you have to push your glutes back, and down, while making sure your knees don't pass your toes. After the physical part is done, now it's time to come up with an exercise, and diet plan to follow.

After consistently working out, and dieting for a month, we'll re-asses to see the client's progression using their prior stats, and pictures. If the goal was reached we'll continue the program with some minor adjustment. But if the goal wasn't reached we would have to take a deeper look as to why it wasn't reached. Especially, if they stuck to the program.

Let's take a look at some of the factors that can play a role in not getting to your fitness goals.

- **Not sticking to the program**
- **Being impatient**
- **Health issues**
- **Giving up**

NOT STICKING TO THE PROGRAM

When it comes to getting clients to stick to a program, this can be difficult for any fitness professional for a lot of reasons. Most clients are not ready mentally, to stick to a long term program. So I always work on their mental first. One question I always ask is "How bad do you want to reach your fitness goal, on a scale of 1 to 10?" Most say 10 but a few say lower because they want to be realistic about their fitness goals, knowing they're not 100% committed.

The people who are not 100% committed will say "I'm going to "try" to stick to the program" my answer to that is "to try is to fail" and here's why. If you tell me "I'm going to "try" to work out, and eat healthy, and for some reason you don't. You can always come back and say "I didn't say I was going to do it. I said I was going to "try" and honestly I'm not mad about it because "to try is to fail." You're either going to do it or not. It's that simple. The "try" in this case is code for it's highly likely it won't get done.

BEING IMPATIENT

Wanting results too fast is a major issue that I've experienced with some clients. During some of my fitness assessments a client would ask, can I lose 30 pounds in a month? As a fitness professional, it's my job to let clients know that while it's possible, it's not healthy, to lose weight that fast. If a person manages to lose 30 pounds in a month, most of that weight loss would come from muscle mass. The draw back to that is, when you lose muscle mass, you actually lower your metabolic rate. And when you lower your metabolic rate you're actually lowering your metabolism. Case in point I've had people tell me that they have lost up to 30 pounds in a month. So, I'd ask, "How did you do it? 90% of the people would say I ran or walked every day, and ate good foods. Then I'd ask, did you gain the weight back? Some people would say yeah, and even more weight. So my next question would be, "did you add any strength training with that program?" Most said no. Then I'd say, you know most of that weight loss came from muscle mass, and because you lost muscle mass you actually lowered your metabolic rate, making it easy for you to gain back the weight.

The problem with this approach is that the focus is on weight loss, and not changing body composition, body fat to muscle ratio. Body composition is way more important than weight loss. Because you can weigh the same, and look different depending on your body composition.

Example, if someone weighs 150 pounds with a 25% muscle mass, and 35% body fat, this person actually has more body fat than muscle mass. So because their muscle mass is low, their metabolic rate is low. Making it easier to store body fat. The other example is someone weighing 150 pounds with a 40% muscle mass and 12% body fat. This person metabolic rate is burning calories more efficiently, because they have a high metabolic rate, because of the amount of muscle mass they have. The ultimate goal on your weight loss journey is to burn fat, and build muscle. And this takes time.

After a month of training a client, I would re-assess them to see how they're progressing. If the weight didn't change, most would be upset, but I would reassure them that it's bigger than the weight loss, and let's see what the body fat to muscle ratio is. I would explain to them that when someone adds muscle while burning fat, and still maintain the same weight that's actually good. Because they're raising their metabolic rate, which will help them burn more calories throughout the day, and help them get rid of the body fat.

Some clients would tell me their clothes fit a little loose now. That's when I'd say, "see it's bigger than losing weight, you want to focus on changing your body composition first." Weight loss takes time. I've trained clients who lost up to 100 pounds, the process took over a year. When it comes to the people who want "overnight success" I'd ask, how long did it take to gain the weight? And I would hear, a year or 2. So I'd say reverse that process. If it took a year to gain, then think of losing it in a year. I always tell my clients that they have to be comfortable with delayed gratification and have the willingness to make sacrifices. Their level of commitment will determine how fast they will reach their goal.

HEALTH ISSUES

Several health issues can hinder someone's fitness goals. When I get to this part of the assessment my job is to find out if there are any health issues that I need to know about, before we can start an exercise program. And if there are any issues, their doctor will have to approve them starting an exercise program. Most of the common issues are

- **Diabetes**
- **Arthritis**
- **Heart disease**
- **Thyroid disease**

When it comes to diabetes, this disease is heredity, and also preventable. This is where managing your diet comes into play. If you keep your blood sugar low, and exercise regularly, this disease is manageable.

With arthritis, regular exercise can help reduce pain, and help maintain strength around the joints, and reduce joint stiffness.

Regular exercise can help improve your heart condition. Heart disease is also preventable, and reversible, if you follow a good nutritional, and exercise program.

Hypothyroidism is a deficiency of the thyroid hormone that can disrupt such things as heart rate, body temperature, and all aspects of metabolism. Hypothyroidism is mostly preventable in older women.

FITNESS AND FINANCE

GIVING UP

Why do people give up on their fitness goals? The number one reason is delayed gratification. Everyone wants results now, and if they don't get results in the time they feel is right, they'll just stop, thinking it's not working. Losing 30 pounds in a month is not healthy. The healthy way to lose weight is to lose about 2 pounds per week. So in a month 8 pounds of weight loss is good, and healthy for the body. The goal here is to lose body fat while building up your muscle mass. Because muscle weighs more than body fat sometimes, the weight might not go down, but the body fat did, and the muscle mass increased. So this process takes time, and giving up too soon can take you, right back where you started.

As you can see there's so many variables that can discourage someone from starting and maintaining a healthy lifestyle.

I want to tell you a quick story about one of my first clients. While working at a gym in NYC at 23rd and Park Ave. I had the pleasure of training one of my favorite clients, her name is Tiffany. She moved to NYC from the Midwest to work for one of the big banks in the area. Tiffany was about 5'4 with an athletic build but was about 20 pounds over-weight. She didn't like the fact that she gained that weight and wanted to get rid of it. She told me that she was able to maintain her athletic physique through high school and college, but when she moved to NYC she gained 20 pounds out of nowhere. During the assessment I asked her what happened and she said that, because in NYC there is food everywhere and there are so many types of foods to choose from. Believe it or not that wasn't the first time I've heard that from someone. She also mentioned that she goes out with friends and co-workers for happy-hour every weekend. This became her lifestyle living in NYC. She came to me to get on a diet and exercise program so she can lose the 20 pounds and get back into shape like she used to be. My job as her fitness coach was to put together a plan for her, that will help her, lose those 20 pounds. The program consisted of her circuit training with me 3 times per week and she would do 30 minutes of light cardio before breakfast (65% of her max heart rate) every day. And the days she didn't train with me, she would have to do explosive cardio in the afternoon or evening. I put her on a diet plan for her to follow while she was on this weight loss program. When putting the diet plan together I let her know she has to start cooking and meal prepping. No more buying take-out for lunch and dinner. I told her to bring her lunch to work, not only do you know what's in the food, you'll be saving money. As for happy hour I let her know she can still hangout with her friends but be cautious on how much she drinks. We spoke about the importance of portion control. Just because it's healthy doesn't mean you can eat any size portion. I told her she can have one cheat meal per week. That was her program and after about 90 days of consistent training she lossed the 20 pounds and was back to her normal weight. I told her now she has to maintain that weight, so she has to stay active and keep a balanced diet. This is the key to staying healthy.

CHAPTER 3

> *"Everyone needs constant education and training. The more you keep yourself informed, the better honed your instincts and decision making capabilities"*
> Linda Conway

FINANCIAL LITERACY

- The lack of financial literacy cost Americans $415 billion in 2020.
- The average credit card debt in America is $6,270.
- Around 40% of Americans have less than $300 in savings.
- Only 30% of Americans have a long-term financial plan.
- The average US household's median income was $78,500 in 2020.
- A staggering 63% of Americans had their personal finances affected by the Covid-19 pandemic.
- Some 44% of Americans expect their finances to improve in 2021.

The lack of money management knowledge may cost you your financial health. According to the NFEC study, the average US citizen lost $1,634 in 2020 because of insufficient personal finance understanding. Even more concerning is the fact that the data represents an increase from the 2018 and 2019 surveys, when Americans lost $1,230 and $1,279, on average.

The definition of financial literacy is the possession of the set of skills, and knowledge that allows an individual to make informed, and effective decisions with all their financial resources, and also the ability to understand, and effectively use various financial skills including personal finance, budgeting and investing. Acquiring financial literacy is the key to financial freedom. Learning, and applying how to manage your finances is very important if you plan on becoming financial free. So what does financial freedom look like. That's when your income can maintain your lifestyle without you having to lift a finger.

One of the books I read on financial literacy was "The Truth About Money" by Ric Edelman. I was introduced to this book by one of my clients I was training at the gym on Park ave. Her name was Jessica and she was from Colombia in South America. She was a college student studying finance at Baruch college. We would talk about her studies in finance during our training sessions, and what she was currently studying at the moment. One day she asked me if I ever read the book "The truth about money" I told her I never heard of it. She told me that was one of the books they were studying in her finance class. She told me the details of the book, so when I got my break from work, I walked down to Barnes and Noble on 17th and Park ave and bought the book. What I love about this book is it breaks down finances from A-Z. Everything from budgeting to estate planning.

FINANCIAL MANAGEMENT

The first thing I want to talk about is managing your income. When it comes to income we can break it down to daily, weekly, monthly, and yearly. This is the first step in tracking how much income you have coming in. Most people I know get paid on a bi-weekly system. When you get paid like this, you have to budget your money so you don't run out before the next paycheck. Also known as living paycheck, to paycheck. Depending on your financial situation this can be tough especially if you're relying on one source of income. Living a lifestyle within your means is very important if you plan on becoming financially free. It is very important that you use your work income to work towards financial freedom. If you don't you'll be working all your life.

We all like nice things, but sometimes we have to think on a deeper level when we decide to make a purchase. Think about this for a minute. The current federal minimum wage is $7.25. Let's take $7.25 times 40 hours a typical work week, and you get $290. That's one week of work. The average cost for a pair of Jordans or Yeezys are over $200. I'm sure you have seen people waiting in long lines for hours just to purchase a pair. When it comes time to make this purchase you have to ask yourself. Are these sneakers worth a week worth of work? Not to mention the time you'll have to wait on the line to get a pair.

In the book "Money master the game" by Tony Robbins stated, "no matter what, always pay yourself first." We tend to pay everyone else before we pay ourselves. There are several ways to pay yourself first, you can have the funds come out of your check straight to your IRA or 401K accounts. Or you can have it go straight to a personal investment account or savings account. You don't only want to work for money, at some point you have to make that money work for you. Start saving, and investing in the future, this is very important, and it must be done sooner than later.

Now let's talk about all those people we tend to pay first. We all have fixed expenses that must be paid monthly. Even during the covid-19 pandemic your fixed expenses had to be paid every month, whether you were working or not. Our biggest monthly fixed expense is housing. Whether you bought a house or renting an apartment you'll have to pay a mortgage or rent to stay where you're living. A general rule is that you don't want to spend more than 30 percent of your monthly income on housing. And that's because you'll have other monthly fixed expenses to pay for. Even if your house is paid for, you'll still have to pay property taxes every year.

Now let's talk about the monthly expenses associated with your housing. We need electricity for our lights, computer, fridge, AC, and TV. That's a monthly fixed expense that must be paid every month. The last thing we want is to be in a house with no electricity. Oh and if you have a computer you'll need an internet provider which is another monthly expense.

Next is transportation. If you live in New York City, you may not need a car, but you'll need a metrocard to ride the subway and buses. A monthly metro card is around $130 per month. For the people who have vehicles, if you're leasing or financing that's a monthly fixed expense that must be paid monthly, if not the repo man will be coming around to repossess the vehicle.

Another fixed monthly expense is car insurance. You do not want to get caught driving around without car insurance. It will end badly for you.

Next up is your phone bill which is due monthly. We all need to communicate with one another so having an active phone is important. Credit cards are another fixed expense, if you're carrying a balance on your card. Also on the list are loans especially student loans.

Finally, I want to mention the last two insurances which are very important to have. If you have a family or not you need to have life insurance, and health insurance. God forbid something happens to you and you don't have neither. These are the main fixed expenses most adults have. Some people have more or less depending on their financial situation. But we have to pay these fixed expenses monthly year over year. With so much money going out, how do we get to save? One thing you have to do as mentioned before pay yourself first.

SAVE 10% OF YOUR INCOME

Here is one of the first rules I learned about personal finances. Pay yourself first! Like I said earlier, we are not living to work hard and pay our hard earned money to someone else and not pay ourselves. The way I pay myself first is I'll take out $50 a week and put it in my investment account. With that $50 I'll buy some stocks. Now what I just did was put that $50 to work. In order to become financially free you have to make your money work for you, instead of just working for money. In a month I would have put in $200 and by the end of the year that account would have an extra $2,400. With the right stock picks that $2,400 could potential double. This is why you have to pay yourself first, so you can have funds to create for an emergency fund, invest, and to save for retirement.

BUDGETING

What is budgeting? It's a simple way to balance your expenses and income. Trimming the fat so to speak. Keeping track of your expenses daily, weekly, and monthly will help you see where you can cut some expenses. Here are a few expenses that are not fixed, and can be eliminated from your expenses.

1. Things like useless subscriptions that are taken out of your account monthly. When signing up for free trials be sure to cancel before the trial date is up. This is a big trap plenty of people get caught up in. These companies are relying on you forgetting to cancel so they can charge you. Beware.

2. Partying every weekend, and going out to dinners. While hanging out with friends and family is needed. But if you're not in a financial position to hangout you should put it off until you can.
3. Unnecessary shopping for things you don't need at the moment. We all have things we want and need, but if it's not something you need for survival, it wouldn't be wise to buy something that you can put off for another time.

Once you cut the "fat" you can use those funds to create an emergency fund. You can set up an account just for this. The purpose of this account is for, if an emergency happens you have the funds available to take care of the problem. Here's something else you can do with those funds, you can invest in easy to liquid assets. Stocks are easy to liquidate. The good thing about stocks is, if you pick the right ones your money can grow over time. We'll go over investing in the stock market later.

WAYS TO INCREASE YOUR INCOME

If you plan on getting out of the rat race, and becoming financially free you'll have to increase your income. It's easier said than done. One of the things you can do to increase your income is get another job, known as a side hustle. If you live in a big city like New York City, it is difficult to live on one source of income. The cost of living is very high and in most cases, one stream of income can't cover the living expenses. The good thing is there are plenty of side hustles you can do to increase your income. One side hustle some of my friends would do was post mates, and Uber eats. Both companies are food delivery companies. Remember my friend Tony who was behind on rent and used his vehicle to increase his income. If you have a vehicle and have some down time you can make an extra $400-$500 per week. Whether it's Uber, Lyft or any other delivery service. This is a great side hustle you can do if you have a vehicle. By utilizing your vehicle to help you increase your income, that vehicle is now an asset not a liability anymore. There are plenty of other ways to increase your income. You can start a business, provide a service, you can sell on ebay and Amazon and invest in the stock market. The point is you have to increase your income to become financially free.

GETTING RID OF BAD DEBT (TRIMMING THE FAT)

Now that you have some extra income it would be wise to start to clear all debt. Student loans, credit cards, mortgage, and car notes to name a few. The thing that hurts with this kind of debt is the interest rates you have to pay on the loans, and credit cards. All of these carry high interest rates that will keep you in debt longer. The goal here is to clear them as fast as you can, and don't get back in debt! The last thing you want to do is default on one of these loans or credit cards, that would impact your credit score negatively, and hurt you in the future if you apply for a loan again. I've fallen to the trap of getting a loan, and credit cards. I have to say it's hard to get ahead financially when you have these types of debt. For me it feels like weight, I can't get rid of it. Month after month, and year after year, I'm paying on something that I used a long time ago. This is the trap to keep you poor, and a slave to these companies. The only reason you should go into debt is if that debt has a potential to bring in an income.

UNDERSTANDING CREDIT AND CREDIT SCORE

Credit is part of your financial power. It will help you to get the things you need, like a loan for a car or a credit card, this will be based on your credit worthiness. Having a good credit score will help you get the best interest rates. Working to improve your credit worthiness is a part of becoming financially free and wealthy. While cash is King, credit is Queen!

Earlier in the book I told you about how my friend Tony sacrificed paying his rent to instead pay off his outstanding bad debt. He made that sacrifice because he knows how important it is to have good credit. And because of that sacrifice, he still has good credit to this day. Cash is King but credit is Queen. If you play chess you'll understand this. The Queen can move all over the board and is the most powerful piece on the board, while the King can only move one space at a time, and the Queen's job is to protect the King. When talking about credit, the Queen can get you things the King can't because cash the King is limited in his moves. Think about this, if you have over $10,000 in cash to buy, say a car. That purchase has to get reported to the IRS because it was over $10,000 in cash. Now if you make that same purchase with credit, the IRS would not need to know about that purchase. Your credit, the Queen is used for so many things you may not even realize. You can be denied an apartment if you have bad credit even if you have the cash the King to pay for it. You can do much more with your credit, the Queen than you can do with cash, the King. Not to mention your credit can get you cash. Whatever you do, make sure to protect your credit score by all means. This is a very important piece of the puzzle for you to build wealth. It would be wise to sign up for a credit monitoring agency, because identity theft is on the rise. You want to also make sure you do routine check ups on your credit report to make sure you don't have anything negative impacting your credit score.

Why is credit so important? When it comes to big purchases like a home, business or a car your credit worthiness is very important to the lender. The lender needs to know you're capable of paying back the loan with interest. So having a credit history is where they will look to see your worthiness. That's why it's important to start your credit history early. And having no credit history is just like having bad credit. You will not get a loan with a good interest rate. So what will determine your interest rate on your loan, is your credit score. Here is a snapshot of the ranges according to the FICO scores.

- **Poor credit: 300-579**
- **Fair credit: 580-669**
- **Good credit: 670-739**
- **Very good credit: 740-799**
- **Excellent credit: 800-850**

Having a good credit score shows lenders, landlords and employers that you are responsible at paying your debts. In this day and age your credit score can affect whether you get an apartment. Some landlords check your credit worthiness to see if they will rent you an apartment. If you live in New York City like me, they will do a credit check before renting you an apartment. Your creditworthiness can also affect you in getting a job. Some employers run a credit check before hiring some employees. So in order to get to financial freedom you have to establish good credit.

How to build good credit? If you want a good credit score, you need to understand how to build credit.

Your FICO credit score is made up of the following five factors:

- **Payment history: 35 percent**
- **Credit utilization: 30 percent**
- **Length of credit history: 15 percent**
- **Credit mix: 10 percent**
- **Recent credit inquiries: 10 percent**

Your payment history makes up 35% of your score. So if you have no history or a short payment history then this will affect your score the most.

Next is credit utilization which makes up 30% of your score. This is how much of your credit is being utilized. Having a high utilization negatively impacts your credit score. It's good to have under 30%

utilization on all credit cards. This means lower interest and better credit score.

Length of history. This makes up 15% of your credit score. Like I said earlier, it's good to start your credit history early. The reason for this is to show that you're responsible for paying debt over the long term. When you get a loan for a home it may be a 30 year loan, or a car can be a 5 year loan.

Having a credit mix is to show you have different types of debt. This makes up 10% of your credit score. Credit cards, car loans and personal loans are different types of debt. This shows you have different types of debt and are able to manage them.

And last inquiries. This makes up 10% of your credit score. This is to show lenders how many loans you've applied for in the past 2 years. Having too many inquiries within 2 years will negatively impact your score. You want to apply for loans when necessary. Inquiries stay on your credit report for 25 months. This has recently been updated in 2020. In the past it would stay on your credit report for 24 months. Once your credit is intact you can move on to investing in the stock market.

INVESTING IN THE STOCK MARKET

Here's the reasons why you should be invested in the stock market. Inflation and compound interest! What is inflation? It's the cost of goods, and services rising in price. If you currently have $1,000 sitting in your bank account for over a year you'll gain, maybe a dollar in interest. With the rate of inflation that $1,000 is now $950. So you actually lose money by not having your money somewhere that would give you a higher return on interest. Now, take that same $1,000 at the start of 2020 and put it in the S&P 500 index fund, you would have gotten a 16% return, and would have $1,160 in your account today. That's how you make your money work for you. So being invested in the stock market, will help to beat inflation in more than one way.

Thanks to today's technology you don't need a stock broker to invest your money in the stock market. But, if you don't have time to look up stocks you like, you can hire a broker who can do it for you, but for a fee. I personally put some money in a Titan account in September, and it's up 16% so far. So you don't have to manage your money yourself. The key here is that you're making your money work for you. I've read that you have to look at your money like little soldiers going out to get more soldiers every day. Using a fund management like Titan is good, but there are other ways to invest in the stock market. You have trading platforms like TD Ameritrade, Webull, Robinhood, E-Trade, M-1, and if you have an IRA account with your bank you can use that to invest.

Some of these platforms have paper trading which you can use to practice, until you become confident enough to use real money. The only problem I have with paper trading is you're not using your hard earned money to make these trades, so there is no emotional attachment to a paper trading account. But, your hard earned money you worked hours at a job for will make you more cautious when you start to make trades. Paper trading is good for you to learn how to use the platform to start making trades. Once you've learned how to use the platform, you can start looking at which investment tool you want to use. There are plenty of ways to invest in the stock market. You have index funds, ETF's, stocks, bonds, mutual funds and more.

When it comes to investing you want to start early and here's why. If you start early, you can take advantage of compound interest. What is compound interest? According to wikipedia Compound interest is the addition of interest to the principal sum of a loan or deposit, or in other words, interest on interest. It is the result of reinvesting interest, rather than paying it out, so that interest in the next period is then earned on the principal sum plus previously accumulated interest. Compound interest is standard in finance and economics. Here is how you can make it work for you.

Say your initial investment was $5,000 at age 20, and you put in $500 every month for 25 years at an interest rate of 10%-15% at age 45 you would have $644,255 in your account with the help of compound interest. Let's put it in perspective by just adding the investment without compound interest. $5,000+$500 times 12 months is $6,000 times 25 years= $150,000+$5,000= $155,000. Let's take $644,255-$155,000=$489,255. So you basically made almost a half a million dollars on compound interest alone. While it's never too late to start, earlier is better. I don't even know where it would have been if you waited until 65 years old. One thing for sure you'd be a millionaire.

Here's how I got started in investing in the stock market. In 2006 a friend of mine came to me one day, and said, hey Tre I'm doing a class on how to trade in the stock market. My initial response was I'm not trying to do that, and lose my money. The next thing he said was, I'll show you how to make money whether the market goes up or down. After he said that, it sparked my interest because I needed to know how you can make money, if the stock market is going down. The class he was teaching was how to trade the S&P 500 e-mini futures. After the first class I became fascinated with trading, because I didn't know you could trade without actually buying a stock. I bought books on how to trade futures, and books on how to read candlestick charts, watch CNBC every day and read the Wall street journal daily. I learned how to be a trader before learning how to be an investor. The draw back to that was I was looking at stocks as trades instead of long term investments.

To this day, I'm thankful for my friend for introducing me on how to trade in the stock market. So I hope you noticed, I said trade the stock market not invest. Just to clarify, these are 2 different ways to play the stock market. The quick example is an investor is someone looking for long term growth in their investment, and a trader is looking for a quick return on their investment. When you first get started you want to be an investor first. So you can start to learn price action, read charts and educate yourself as you go. Then later if you want, you can start to make trades. Once you learn, you'll be able to get good returns on your investments, if you do it right. All you have to do is buy stocks at a low price and sell it high.

Back in 2013 me and one of my co-workers were having a conversation in the break room about how to increase our income. At that point I mentioned that I know how to trade in the futures market specifically the S&P 500 e-mini. He was hype about it and suggested we start a company and trade under that company. So we formed an LLC T&H Holdings. We reached out to a discount brokerage in Chicago called Apex Futures and we traded under that brokerage firm. We funded the account and were ready to rock and roll. The good thing was that they had an app we could download and trade from. Also you can paper trade.

Let me break down how the S&P 500 e-mini works. Each point on the S&P 500 e-mini is equivalent to $50. Each point is broken down into quarters, so each quarter or "tick" is equivalent to $12.50. Our first week of trading we made $1,000 and we did this while training our clients. We were excited to see such gains in a week. As we were training and trading, some of our trades would go bad and by the time we would notice, we would have a big loss. The thing about the S&P 500 e-mini, you can be up $500 in 2 minutes, and down that same amount in 2 minutes. So because we couldn't manage the account, we decided to shut it down. When trading, any trader will tell you that you have to watch your trades. So we moved on from that and focused on investing, since you don't have to watch your stock every day.

I've made several good trades in 2020, but I'll talk about this one trade I did in my IRA account. On October 12th. I bought 100 shares in stock symbol CBAT for $300, so it was trading at $3 per share. On November 16th it was trading at over $11. Before the close of the day I sold my 100 shares at $1,088 for over 300% return in a little over a month. For a profit of $788. Today that stock is trading at $4.68 more than half of where I sold it. That was a trade, not a long term investment. But I also have stocks that I am invested in for the long term like the airline industry, tech stocks and electric vehicles. Because of the covid-19 pandemic the airline industry has been hit hard, and so has their stock prices. Currently these stocks are at a discount, because not too many are traveling right now. But once it picked up, so will their stock prices.

I want to take a little time to explain how you can make money by having a stock price go down. I used "options" to make this trade. With options you have calls (means buy) and you have puts (means sell). I recently got a put (sell) option on a stock symbol NKLA. It was trading at around $27, and I put a strike price of $17.50. So I felt like this stock will go down to $17.50 within a given time frame. I paid $115 for 1 contract which was going to expire in 3 weeks. The thing about options is your trade starts to add value once the price is moving in your direction. 2 weeks into the trade the stock dropped past my strike price to $16.50. I sold it at $365 for a $250 profit. That was actually my first option play for the year. As you can see you can utilize the stock market to make your money work for you. This is a big part when it comes to financial freedom.

CHAPTER 4

> *"Nothing can stop a person with the right mental attitude from achieving their goal; nothing on earth can help a person with the wrong mental attitude"*
> **Thomas Jefferson**

DIET AND EXERCISE

In the US in 2017, 18.66% of all deaths are attributed to heart disease, whereas another 6.03% and 6.67% are caused by strokes and lung cancer, respectively.

Unhealthy eating and lifestyle habits are the leading cause of death in the US, as the latest unhealthy eating statistics show. Yet, the current data also shows some promise with a steady decline in the number of cases in respect to last year's figures with a 1.39% annual change in heart failure, 0.28% in strokes, and a 0.095% decrease in terminal lung cancer cases.

Source: Institute for Health Metrics and Evaluation

Diet related diseases like diabetes, cardiovascular disease, high blood pressure, and obesity are a major problem in our society. These diet related diseases have a big impact on our society and economy.

Because of these health issues we pay higher taxes to cover the cost of Medicare and Medicaid. Type 2 diabetes cost about $500 billion annually. A change in the diet and living a healthy lifestyle could dramatically cut this cost. When it comes to type 2 diabetes, things like blindness, can start to set in, kidney failure, and limb amputation. These issues could be avoided with a proper balanced diet and exercise program.

Disease	Cost
Diabetes	$245 Billion
Cancer	$216.6 Billion
Coronary heart disease	$204.4 Billion
Obesity	$190 Billion
High blood pressure	$46.4 Billion
Stroke	$36.5 Billion
Osteoporosis	$19 Billion

Source: Center for Science in the Public Interest

When it comes to your body fat, for women and men it should be at a certain percentage range depending on your age. The goal here is to keep your body fat as low as possible.

Interpreting the Body Fat Percentage Result

Gender	Age	Low (−)	Normal (0)	High (+)	Very High (++)
Female	20-39	< 21.0	21.0 - 32.9	33.0 - 38.9	≥ 39.0
	40-59	< 23.0	23.0 - 33.9	34.0 - 39.9	≥ 40.0
	60-79	< 24.0	24.0 - 35.9	36.0 - 41.9	≥ 42.0
Male	20-39	< 8.0	8.0 - 19.9	20.0 - 24.9	≥ 25.0
	40-59	< 11.0	11.0 - 21.9	22.0 - 27.9	≥ 28.0
	60-79	< 13.0	13.0 - 24.9	25.0 - 29.9	≥ 30.0

BODY FAT RANGE FOR WOMEN AND MEN

Example women ages 20-39 years old "low" 21% and under. That means you have a low body fat percentage. "Normal body fat" is 21%-32.9% that's the body percentage most people in that age range have. "High body fat" is 33%-38.9% for this age range. "Very high body fat" is 39% and above for this age range. Women with an age range from 40-59 years old fall in a different category. "Low body fat" is 23% and under. "Normal body fat" is 23%-33.9%, "high body fat is 34%-39.9% and "very high body fat is 40% and more. Women with an age range from 60-79 years old fall in a different category. "Low body fat" is 24% and under. "Normal body fat" is 24%-34.9%, "high body fat" is 36%-41.9% and "very high body fat" is 42 and above.

For men the body fat percentages should be within a certain range depending on your age. Example men ages 20-39 "Low body fat" is 8% or less, "Normal body fat" is 8%-19.9%, "high body fat" is 20%-24.9%, "very high body fat" is 25% and above for this age range. Men with an age range from 40-59 years old fall in a different category. "Low body fat" is 11% and under. "Normal body fat" is 11%-21.9%, "high body fat is 22%-27.9% and "very high body fat is 28% and more. Men with an age range from 60-79 years old fall in a different category. "Low body fat" is 13% and under. "Normal body fat" is 13%-24.9%, "high body fat" is 25%-29.9% and "very high body fat" is 30 and above.

Interpreting the Skeletal Muscle Percentage Result

Gender	Age	Low (−)	Normal (0)	High (+)	Very High (++)
Female	18-39	< 24.3	24.3 - 30.3	30.4 - 35.3	≥ 35.4
	40-59	< 24.1	24.1 - 30.1	30.2 - 35.1	≥ 35.2
	60-80	< 23.9	23.9 - 29.9	30.0 - 34.9	≥ 35.0
Male	18-39	< 33.3	33.3 - 39.3	39.4 - 44.0	≥ 44.1
	40-59	< 33.1	33.1 - 39.1	39.2 - 43.8	≥ 43.9
	60-80	< 32.9	32.9 - 38.9	39.0 - 43.6	≥ 43.7

SKELETAL MUSCLE RANGE FOR WOMEN AND MEN

Skeletal muscle is very important in health and fitness. The goal here is to have a high muscle percentage. For one the more muscle you have, the more efficiently your body burns calories. Two your muscles are stronger to deal with every day tasks. You should be at a certain muscle percentage range for your age.

Example women ages 18-39 "low muscle" 24% and under, "normal muscle" 24.3%-30.1%, "high muscle" 30.4%-35-3% and "very high muscle" 35.4%. Women ages 40-59 fall in a different category, "low muscle" 24.1% and under, "normal muscle" 24.1%-30.1%, "high muscle" 30.2%-35-1% and "very high muscle" 35.2%. Women ages 60-80 fall in a different category. "low muscle" 23.9% and under, "normal muscle" 23.9%-29.9%, "high muscle" 30%-34.9% and "very high muscle" 35%.

For men example ages 18-39 "low muscle" 33.3% and under, "normal muscle" 33.3%-39.9%, "high muscle" 39.4%-44.% and "very high muscle" 44.1%. Men ages 40-59 fall in a different category, "low muscle" 33.1% and under, "normal muscle" 33.1%-39.1%, "high muscle" 39.2%-43.8% and "very high muscle" 43.9%. Men ages 60-80 fall in a different category. "low muscle" 32.9% and under, "normal muscle" 32.9%-39.9%, "high muscle" 39%-43.6% and "very high muscle"43.7%.

According to the New England Journal of Medicine, research found the number of adults who are projected to have obesity will rise over the next decade. Specifically, they estimate the share of U.S.A adults with obesity is expected to reach 48.9% in 2030, up from an estimated 42% in 2020. The BMI is used to determine your weight class. If your BMI is under 21 you're considered underweight. If your BMI is 22 to 25 you're considered normal weight. If your BMI is over 25 but under 30, you're considered overweight and 30 or more is obese.

Interpreting the BMI Result

BMI	BMI (Designation by the WHO)	BMI Classification Bar (- 0 + ++)	BMI Rating
Less than 18.5	- (Underweight)		7.0 - 10.7 10.8 - 14.5 14.6 - 18.4
18.5 or more and less than 25	0 (Normal)		18.5 - 20.5 20.6 - 22.7 22.8 - 24.9
25 or more and less than 30	+ (Overweight)		25.0 - 26.5 26.6 - 28.2 28.3 - 29.9
30 or more	++ (Obese)		30.0 - 34.9 35.0 - 39.9 40.0 - 90.0

BMI RANGE

The main cause of obesity is eating too much, and moving too little. If you eat too much, and don't use the calories consume regularly, any extra calories that is not used get stored as body fat.

Body fat and bad debt have something in common. We all don't want it, and want to get rid of it fast. But it's not that easy, it takes patience and a lot of work. This is where you have to except delayed gratification. It's a process. You have to start by creating a diet, and exercise program that will help get you in good physical health. First thing that has to be done is changing your mindset about food. Instead living to eat, you have to eat to live. Start eating foods that's going to nourish your body. Not only do you want to eat healthy you want to have a timeline on when to eat. I give all my clients a nutritional guideline to follow. That breaks down what to eat from breakfast to dinner. When it comes to losing weight, what you feed your body is very important.

Visceral fat is fat that wraps around your abdominal organs deep inside your body. You can't always feel it or see it. In fact, you may have a pretty flat tummy and still have visceral fat.

Interpreting the Visceral Fat Level Result

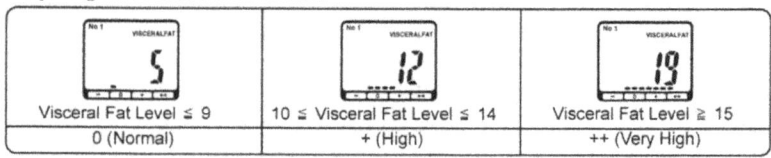

VISCERAL FAT LEVELS

Stay away from foods high in sugar, saturated fats, trans fat, fried foods, process foods, and high starch foods. The goal is to focus on low energy carbs like veggies, fruits, and lean cut meats. Portion size is also very important in losing fat. Depending on the rate of your metabolism, keeping your portion sizes small per meal should be the goal. With a combination of protein, low energy carbs, and healthy fats.

To preserve muscle mass you have to get at least 20-30 grams of protein each meal and snack. By preserving, and adding muscle mass, you're raising your metabolism so your body burns calories more efficiently. This is why you'll need to get on an exercise program and diet plan, so you can build muscle, then you'll burn more calories daily.

MACRONUTRIENTS CARBS, PROTEIN AND FATS

According to Harvard Health letter, eating breakfast regularly has been linked to lower risk of obesity, diabetes, and heart disease. But this seem to be the meal most people that I've trained have the hardest time with. The main reason is, they can't eat that early. My solution for them is, if you can't eat your nutrients that early, then drink it. Make a shake or smoothie that's balanced with protein, carbs, and fats. This is even more important if you exercise in the morning. If you don't nourish your body before you exercise you run the risk of feeling lightheaded, lethargic, and passing out. When it comes to nourishing your body according to the Mayo Clinic, you want to get about 45% to 65% of your daily calories from healthy carbs especially if you exercise.

CARBOHYDRATES

Each gram of carbohydrate contains 4 calories. But not all carbohydrate are created equal. Focusing on low glycemic carbs like, sweet potatoes, spinach, green bean, asparagus, steel cut oatmeal, and bananas to name a few. These carbs are good to eat throughout the day. When you eat low glycemic carbs it doesn't spike your insulin like high glycemic carbs, like sugar, white bread, and white potatoes. The only time you want to eat high glycemic carbs is after exercising. When your body needs to replenish its glycogen stores.

PROTEIN

Each gram of protein contains 4 calories. Protein is very important when it comes to building, and maintaining muscle mass. The Recommend Dietary Allowance (RDA) for protein in non-exercising individuals is 0.8 grams of protein per kilogram of body weight. For individuals who exercise regularly its recommended to have 1.2-1.8 grams of protein per kilogram of body weight. The main reason why your body needs more protein when exercising is because of the breakdown of muscle tissue that has to repair itself after a strenuous workout. When the muscle tissue has repaired its self, it becomes stronger, and bigger. And it also helps build up your metabolic rate, known as metabolism.

FATS

Each gram of fat contains 9 calories. When it comes to fats not all are created equal. There are 3 different types of fats. Monounsaturated, polyunsaturated, and saturated fat.

Monounsaturated fat, this type of fat is found in a variety of foods and oils. Studies show that eating foods rich in monounsaturated fatty acids instead of saturated fats improves blood cholesterol levels, which can decrease your risk of heart disease, and may also help decrease the risk of type 2 diabetes.

Polyunsaturated fat, is found in plants, and animal foods, such as salmon, vegetable oils, and some nuts and seeds.

Saturated fat, It is one of the unhealthy fats, along with trans-fat. These fat's are most often solid at room temperature. Foods like butter, palm, coconut oils, cheese, and red meat have high amounts of saturated fat.

I recommend to my clients to stay away from saturated fats especially if they currently have any of the health issues mentioned above. Having a well-balanced diet is the key to reaching your health and fitness goals. The other part is exercising regularly. The goal here is to make your diet, and fitness a part of your lifestyle.

EXERCISING

In 2008, Federal Physical Activity Guidelines for Americans was released, and the Healthy People 2020 physical activity objectives developed in 2010 reflected these guidelines. From 2008 to 2018, the rate for adults aged 18 years and over who met the guidelines for aerobic physical activity and muscle-strengthening activity increased by 31.9%, from 18.2% to 24.0% (age adjusted), exceeding the Healthy People 2020 target of 20.1%.

In contrast, between 2005–2008 and 2013–2016, the obesity rate among adults aged 20 years and over increased by 13.9%, from 33.9% to 38.6% (age adjusted), while the change in the rate was not statistically significant among youth aged 2–19 years (16.1% in 2005–2008 and 17.8% in 2013–2016).

Starting an exercise program may be one of the best things you can do for your physical health. Physical activity can reduce your risk of chronic disease, improve your balance, and coordination, help you lose weight, and even improve your sleep habits and self-esteem. These are some of the benefits you'll get from adding an exercise program to your lifestyle. Not to mention, less doctor visits, getting off medications, and just feeling good overall especially when other people notice, and compliment you on your progression.

The first thing you want to do is talk to your doctor before starting any exercise program. If you have any preexisting conditions, you'll have to get a waiver from your doctor to start an exercise program. The reason for this is because the fitness coach need to know, do you have any health issues the would put you at risk. Here are some of the health issues that will require a doctor's waiver.

- **Stroke**
- **Metabolic syndrome**
- **High blood pressure**
- **Type 2 diabetes**
- **Depression**
- **Anxiety**
- **Many types of cancer**
- **Arthritis**

If you have any of these issues talk to your doctor first to make sure it's okay to start exercising, and in some cases, the doctor will recommend a modified exercise program.

Once you get started you'll notice a change in your energy levels. Things that would get you tired or winded, will now seem easier to accomplish. One of the exercises, I would have all my clients do is, run or walk the stairs. I would have them do this for a few reasons.

1) The cardiovascular effect. I would use this as cardio in between each set. Most clients hated it and dread it. But after a few weeks, they would tell me that they noticed that they don't winded going up the stairs anymore. That's when they would start to appreciate running the stairs.
2) The functional effect. Not everyone can go up and down the stairs efficiently. For some they have to learn how to walk up and down the stairs properly.

When you start your fitness journey you must strive to get at least 150 minutes a week of moderate exercise activity or 75 minutes a week of vigorous physical activity, or a combination of moderate and vigorous activity. The guidelines suggest that you spread this exercise throughout the week. I prefer 3 times a week of strength training with cardiovascular training in between days. Example; Monday, Wednesday and Friday are strength training days, and Tuesday and Thursday are cardio days. Saturday and Sunday are rest days.

Getting started requires little to no equipment. You can use your body weight to start your program. And I highly recommend that you master your body weight before you move on to weights. You want to make sure your joints and ligaments are strong enough to handle the weights.

You can get a pair of dumbbells. Which is easy to store and portable. You can work out indoors or outdoors.

Also portable are resistance bands. Resistance bands are easy on the joints, and gives you variable resistance. There are different types and styles to chose from.

There are so many fitness equipment out now, that there is no reason why you can't get started. Not to mention since the covid-19 pandemic, online training has become popular. So you can work out from the comfort of your own home.

The first person I trained that loss 100 pounds was Jack. I remember the day Jack came in for his fitness assessment. We sat down and did his PAR-Q, then after that, I did his stats, where I took his weight, BMI, body fat and muscle mass. He weighed 300 pounds and his BMI was over 40. I explained to him where he was at physically and told him that he was obese according to the BMI chart. When he heard that he was obese, he said that's what triggered him to get started on this weight loss journey. He later confess to me that he had no intentions on hiring a fitness coach, but when he saw that he was considered obese, he knew he had to take action.

I put together a monthly exercise and diet plan for him to follow. In the first month he loss 20 pounds. Then a next 30 pounds, and in 90 days he loss 50 pounds! When we first got started we had a bet, he told me if I can help to get him down 100 pounds he would buy me sushi. At that time I never had sushi, so he wanted to be the first person to introduce it to me. After about 6 months Jack was looking like a new person. One day he walked by me in the gym and I didn't know it was him. When he came out of the locker room I told him, you just walked by me and I didn't even know it was you. He was looking like a new person. Everyone in the gym was congratulating him on his weight loss journey. When he hit his goal he took me out for that sushi liked he promised. When Christmas time came he gave me a card and in the card was a picture of his monthly weight loss progression. I saw shocked because I didn't know he was doing it. And that's why I tell all clients my to take progression pics so they can see their transformation.

The following is the method I use with my clients when they are on their weight loss journey. I require all clients to get a fitness tracker. The reason for having a fitness tracker is so they can keep track of their daily calorie burn. This is important because you have to make sure you're burning more calories than you consume.

I'll give a client two choices between 2% or 3% of their body weight to lose for the month. Once I know which goal they pick, I'll take the weight and divide it by 0.02% or 0.03%. Example 180 pounds divided by 0.03%= 5.4 pounds, that would be the target goal to lose for the month. Then I'll take 5.4 times 3,500 (there is 3,500 calories in 1 pound of fat)= 18,900 that is the total calorie deficit for the month. Now it's time to break it down into a daily calorie deficit, take 18,900 divided by 30 days= 630 calories, you'll have to burn the calories you consume plus your calorie deficit, example; If your resting metabolic rate is 1500. You have to burn 1500+630=2,130. 2,130 is the amount of calories you must burn every day for 30 days to lose 5.4 pounds in 30 days.

I require that clients hit their daily target every day. And if they don't they'll have to make it up somewhere down the line by doing above the daily calorie deficit. Maintaining a consistent calorie deficit will put you on the path to your weight loss goal. Let's not forget, it's not just about weight loss, but also overall physical health.

If you can manage to stay consistent on your physical health, journey you can do the same in personal finance. Just look at personal finances the same way you look at your physical health goals. Both are equally important to your lifestyle. And in my opinion you can't prioritize one over the other.

CHAPTER 5

> *"My favorite things in life don't cost any money. It's really clear that the most precious resource we all have is time"*
> **Steve Jobs**

Now that you have an understanding of the importance of your physical health, and wealth, it's time to create a plan to manage each one into your lifestyle. It's one thing to have the knowledge, but it's nothing without execution. This is where you have to shift your mindset to staying focused on the goals. Because no matter how bad you want it, if you're not ready mentally, it will not happen. This is a major roadblock for a lot of people. And if you're struggling with this, you can find a coach or mentor who will push you through those roadblocks. Not only do you need a coach for your physical health, and wealth, you also need one for your mindset. Mental health is also very important in this process. This can make or break you physically, and financially. Now let's talk about coming up with a plan for you to maintain your health and fitness goals.

MANAGING AND MAINTAINING YOUR HEALTH AND FITNESS

When it comes to your health, and fitness goals, it's best to have a plan to follow. This is something you don't want to freestyle. If you don't have a plan, hire a health, and fitness coach who can put together a plan for you, to reach your goals. The first phase is knowing where you are today, and knowing where you want to be. Example, if your goal is to lose weight you have to figure out how much weight you want to lose. Once you have that number, it's time to come up with a plan for your daily, weekly, and monthly goals. These goals will be both exercise and diet. You'll have to do something every day that will get you to your goals. Strength training three days a week, and cardio three to five days a week is good for overall health. So staying focused, and accepting delayed gratification is the key. Keeping track of your daily calorie deficit is very important. This is where your fitness tracker watch comes in. The way to lose weight if you have to burn more calories than you consume. So sticking to low calorie foods will make this process easier.

Exercising is half the battle, the other half is, what you put in your body. Some people think just because they are exercising that they can eat whatever they want. This should not be the mindset when it comes to physical. Because some foods can cause illness like diabetes, and cardiovascular disease. So eating healthy, and clean is very important to your overall health.

Just like your exercise plan you need one for your diet. It would be a good idea to invest in hiring a dietitian who can come up with a plan for your needs. Remember not everyone can follow the same diet, and get the same results. A lot of factors come in to play here. Things like age, body type, and metabolic rate. Having a dietitian on your team will make things easier. From my experience as a fitness coach this is where most people have a hard time. Because there are so many variables when it comes to the dieting. You have to figure out what kind of foods to eat, the portion size, what times to eat, meal prepping, reading labels, and what to eat when dining out. This can be overwhelming especially if you're just starting out. It's no wonder why most people have a hard time sticking to a diet plan. It requires a lot of work and discipline. One thing you can do to take off some of the load is hire a meal prep service, especially if you don't know how to cook. Not only do they make good foods, it is also well balanced, and you get an actual portion size of each macronutrient, so you don't have to worry about overeating. And there you have it. Putting together a health and fitness plan that will help you reach your physical health goals. With time and patients you'll be on autopilot with your health and fitness goals. Now that you have your physical health plan in order let's work on your wealth. Because health is wealth right?

MANAGING AND MAINTAINING YOUR WEALTH

Just like your physical health you need a plan for your wealth, if you plan on becoming wealthy. Hiring a financial coach is very important in creating a portfolio for your finances. The job of a financial coach is almost the same as a fitness coach or any other coach. Their job is to help you with your short term, and long term financial goals, and to make sure your money, is making you money, and you're not losing money.

The first thing you want to do is figure out your short term and long term financial goals. Short term (1-5 years) financial goals are things like paying off debt, saving an emergency fund, and saving for a down payment on a home. Long term (10-30 years) goals retirement account, paying off your mortgage, and any outstanding debt. This is where you create a plan to manage, and maintain both your short term, and long term financial goals. This is important because you want to retire comfortably without stressing how you'll pay for your current lifestyle.

Your short term financial goals will help you get to your long term financial goals, and shouldn't be taken lightly. Delayed gratification, will have you living comfortably, in your later years in life. So work on these goals as soon as possible.

1) 401k account. If your employer offers a 401k be sure to take advantage of it before you open an IRA, especially if the company matches your contribution. A 401(k) withdraws money from your paycheck, and directly deposits those funds into a retirement account, which is then invested in stocks and bonds. Companies often match a certain percentage of your salary, such as 3%, as long as you contribute to the plan as well. You can contribute to both an IRA and a 401(k) in the same year. However, there are contribution limits for 401(k)s. For 2020 and 2021, you can contribute up to $19,500 per year into a 401(k) or a Roth 401(k). And put your savings on auto-pilot, "Money deposited straight into your retirement account can't be spent elsewhere, and won't be missed. It also helps you maintain discipline with your savings."

2) Paying off debt, bad debt, is like having an anchor on you holding you down from getting to wealth. The goal is to get rid of bad debt, as soon as possible. Doing this will lighten the load on fixed expenses, and save you hundreds if not thousands on interest rate payments. There are two ways to get rid of debt faster. The snowball approach, and avalanche approach. The snowball approach is where you work to pay off the smallest debt, towards the bigger debt. Because this debt is small it will be paid off faster, and

the faster you pay the less interest you'll pay on the debt. Also once it's paid off you'll increase your credit score, and overall credit worthiness. After you finish paying this off the goal is not to get into bad debt ever again. The avalanche approach is different, and it's the flip side to the snowball approach. With this you take the highest interest rate debt, and pay that one down first. Basically, you're clearing the heavy debt to the lightest debt. The benefit of the approach is, you will save a lot on interest, being that this debt has a very high interest rate, so it makes sense to pay this off as soon as possible. Again saving hundreds to thousands of dollars in interest.

3) Pay yourself first, this is so important, and many people don't do it. Especially if you are living paycheck to paycheck, this can be hard. The key here is to have the funds come out of your account before you get it. Having an IRA account or a 401k account is a great way to do this. Your funds will come out automatically, and go to your investment account, and your funds will start to accumulate, and you won't even notice. You also want to save up, an emergency fund. Anything unexpectedly can happen at any time. An example is the covid-19 pandemic. Millions of people lost their jobs, and had to rely on their savings to get by. So, save for that rainy day because you never know when it's going to come.

4) Saving up for a down payment of a home. When it comes to home ownership you have to think smart, and about your financial future. You can buy a one family home, and assume full liability on that home. So the home will be a liability to you, because it's not bringing in any income, and you have to pay a mortgage every month, and all other expenses associated with the home. Or you can buy a two-family

home, live on one side, and rent out the other side. The rent from the other home, should pay for the mortgage or most of it. If you do that, you'll be basically living rent free because someone else is paying the mortgage, and at the same time building equity into the home. After a few years of living there, you can pull some equity from the home to buy another home. And if you want a one family you can get it now, because you have rental income that can help you maintain both mortgages.

These are just a few short term goals you want to have in place so you can work towards your long term goals. Next we'll talk about long term financial goals.

Setting up your long term financial goals will help you get to financial freedom, and help you retire comfortably. Setting up a retirement very early in life will pay off in the long run. If you open an Roth IRA account or have a 401k through your job, you will be setting up for your future. Remember the goal here is to live comfortably, and stress free during retirement. So let's break down the two types of accounts

5) Roth IRA account. According to Investopedia the Roth works differently from traditional IRA accounts. Suppose, you contribute the same $6,000 per year for 40 years to a Roth IRA. You get no immediate tax deduction, but if the Roth IRA grows to $1.6 million (assuming the same 8% annual return). At age 63, you withdraw $50,000 per year. The difference now is that there is no tax due on the Roth withdrawal, because distributions made after retirement are tax-free. In this scenario, you withdraw $50,000, and keep the full amount. In this case, the Roth IRA is clearly the best, and wisest long-term decision when you're in your 20's. Due to the tax benefits of Roth IRAs, 20-somethings,

should seriously consider contributing to one. The Roth can be a wiser long-term choice, even though contributions to a traditional IRA are tax-deductible.

6) Open up an investment account. You can open up an investment account with a few platforms like TD Ameritrade, E-trade and Fidelity. The goal here is to invest in the stock market for long term growth on your money. The stock market has a wide range of asset classes you can invest in, things like traditional stocks, ETFs, index funds, bonds, and mutual funds just to name a few. You want to consistently invest monthly and yearly. By investing in just the S&P 500 index your yearly return could be 8-12% per year. And let's not forget the compound interest you'll gain year after year. After 20-30 years you'll have a good cushion for retirement.

Managing your physical health and wealth can be a challenge if you don't know where to start. This book outlined some key things to help you with physical health and building wealth for the future. But in order to enjoy your life in the future you have to manage and maintain a healthy lifestyle through diet and exercise. The last thing you want, is to become wealthy and can't enjoy it because of illnesses, and other things that will prevent you from enjoying life. So it's time to work towards physical health, and wealth, and live your best life during your retirement years.

ABOUT THE AUTHOR

Tre Fit is a certified NASM CPT/CES and Precision nutrition coach from Brooklyn NY. During his time as a fitness coach he's helped some of his clients lose up to 100 pounds! Back in 2006 Tre was introduced to trading from a friend who taught him how to trade the S&P 500 E-mini futures. Since then Tre has become passionate about personal finances and investing. He has also helped some of his clients learn how to start investing in the stock market and understand the importance of having good credit. Back in 2014 Tre competed in his first NPC fitness competition in men's physique and placed 3rd.

After seeing the correlation between fitness and personal finance he wrote this book on the 2 subjects he is passionate about physical health and wealth.

www.ingramcontent.com/pod-product-compliance
Lightning Source LLC
Chambersburg PA
CBHW060714030426
42337CB00017B/2864